# THINK AND EAT
## YOURSELF
# SMART

## • WORKBOOK •

# THINK AND EAT
## YOURSELF
# SMART

### • WORKBOOK •

### A NEUROSCIENTIFIC APPROACH
### TO A SHARPER MIND AND HEALTHIER LIFE

## DR. CAROLINE LEAF

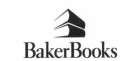

BakerBooks
*a division of Baker Publishing Group*
**Grand Rapids, Michigan**

© 2019 by Caroline Leaf

Published by Baker Books
a division of Baker Publishing Group
PO Box 6287, Grand Rapids, MI 49516-6287
www.bakerbooks.com

Printed in the United States of America

ISBN 978-0-8010-9351-7

Portions of this text taken from *Think and Eat Yourself Smart*, published by Baker Books, 2016

This publication is intended to provide helpful and informative material on the subjects addressed. Readers should consult their personal health professionals before adopting any of the suggestions in this book or drawing inferences from it. The author and publisher expressly disclaim responsibility for any adverse effects arising from the use or application of the information contained in this book.

19  20  21  22  23  24  25        7  6  5  4  3  2  1

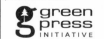

# Contents

# Introduction

We live in a world where the McDonald's sign is more recognizable than the Christian cross, where more and more people suffer from obesity and malnutrition—a world where thousands of people die from preventable lifestyle diseases. Indeed, many of us are unwittingly exposed to foods that affect our physical and mental health, from weight gain and cardiovascular disease to depression and anxiety, which can make us feel like our life is spiraling out of control.

As I discussed in my book *Think and Eat Yourself Smart*, we are facing a global food crisis—something that affects us *all*. Notwithstanding the many ways we have advanced as a civilization, we still have a long way to go, especially when it comes to what we put on our plates and how we treat our environment.

But we cannot change the way we eat if we do not change our thinking. It is important to acknowledge that what we *think* affects what we eat, and what we *eat* affects what we think. To fix our global food crisis, we need to think and eat ourselves smart!

I created this workbook as a guide to help you understand and apply the principles of thinking and eating I outlined in *Think and Eat Yourself Smart*. Each key follows the main themes of the three parts of the book, with a series of questions that will help you understand and apply the information found in the book. Some questions may be repeated or asked in different ways—this is not an error! Repetition and the process of asking, answering, and discussing are integral to cognitive development; it is always important to ask a lot of questions from a variety of perspectives!

# How to Use This Workbook

This workbook is part of a three-part curriculum:

1. The *Think and Eat Yourself Smart* book
2. The *Think and Eat Yourself Smart* DVD
3. The *Think and Eat Yourself Smart* workbook

The DVD and workbook are organized around nine "keys" for a nine-week study. That is sixty-three days, although you can work through the study in more or less time if desired. It takes around twenty-one days to rewire neural pathways and begin building a new way of thinking about your life. It takes an additional forty-two days (two sets of twenty-one days), for a total of sixty-three days, to establish a new habit. Thus, this workbook is designed to help you establish a habit of thinking and learning that will lay the foundation for a healthy life, both mentally and physically.

As you work through the questions in each key, be as specific and honest as you can. Research shows change happens when we use our minds to develop our understanding. Each question will have a section where you can write your answers. If you need more space, you are more than welcome to use a separate journal or notebook—writing down what you think about is essential to learning, so write away!

Once you have completed the questions, there is a discussion section at the end of each key that will draw on different Scripture verses to help you see the connection between science and belief. I would recommend working through the questions and Scripture discussions a second time, after you have completed the workbook, which will help you better understand and apply the principles in *Think and Eat Yourself Smart*. I have used the New Revised Standard Version, as it is a fairly accurate translation of the Bible, both in terms of language and in terms of cultural context. You are welcome to use other translations, or even translate the Scriptures yourself if desired. Shifting between translations will force you to analyze the Scriptures from a variety of different viewpoints, worldviews, and social nuances, which certainly increases mind health! I highly recommend *The Kingdom New Testament* by N. T. Wright, one of the leading New Testament scholars in our world today. Wright's translation pays close attention to the historical context of the New Testament Gospels and letters, allowing the reader to step into the world of the first century CE and truly experience the writings of the early followers of the Messiah. David Bentley Hart recently came out with an incredible, raw, and intimate translation of the New Testament that I highly recommend as well.

At the end of the workbook, there is a recommended reading list for those who wish to dig deeper into the key points I have written about in *Think and Eat Yourself Smart* and this workbook. Many of these sources can be found in the bibliography and notes in *Think and Eat Yourself Smart*, but I have highlighted the most important books and articles and added a few new sources I have researched since writing the book in 2016.

When you begin to follow the guidelines of *Think and Eat Yourself Smart*, your life will begin to change for the better. You will learn how to control what you allow into your head and on your plate, you will discover what is wrong with our current food system, you will learn how to quit this system, and you will learn how to beat it! You are more than capable of taking control of your physical and mental health. You can think and eat yourself smart!

# KEY

# 1

## Prologue

Read pages 13–17 in *Think and Eat Yourself Smart* and watch the key 1 video.

1. *We need to increase our knowledge about food and food practices. We need to improve our shopping and cooking skills. And, most importantly, we need to change our attitudes toward food, health, healing, and nutrition.* Why is this important? How can you improve the way you eat and the way you think about food?

_____

_____

_____

_____

_____

2. *Thinking plays a dominant role in eating.* How so? What role does thinking play in your food choices?

_____

_____

_____

_____

3. *There is always someone new telling us they have the solution to everyone's dietary and/or exercise habits, suggesting that if we don't follow their advice we will surely drop dead.* Have you experienced this in your life? How does this make you feel? Do you think that there is just one way of eating that works for everyone?

_____

_____

_____

_____

4. *It would be much better to understand the fundamentals of eating, the completely entangled relationship between thinking and food, and how our uniqueness spreads throughout our spirit, soul, and body.* Why is this a better way of approaching food than focusing on specific diets or foods? How does this compare to the way you think about and eat food?

_____

_____

_____

_____

5. *I think the fact that we feel we cannot even make our own food choices anymore without the help of an "expert" is a sign of just how broken our food system has become.* Do you agree? If yes, why? If no, why not?

_____

_____

_____

_____

6. *The world we live in desperately needs transformation.* What is wrong with the current food system? Why does it need to be changed?

_____

_____

_____

_____

_____

7. *What exactly is stopping us from avoiding illnesses and premature deaths that are largely preventable? How have our choices led us down this destructive road, away from God's perfect plan for our lives (Jer. 29:11)?* How would you answer these questions? How do you think we can change?

_____

_____

_____

_____

_____

*Think and Eat Yourself Smart* focuses on the state of our current food system. Discuss the following verses in light of this theme.

1. **Romans 12:2.** Do not be conformed to this world, but be transformed by the renewing of your minds, so that you may discern what is the will of God—what is good and acceptable and perfect.

2. **1 Thessalonians 5:23.** May the God of peace himself sanctify you entirely; and may your spirit and soul and body be kept sound and blameless at the coming of our Lord Jesus Christ.

3. **Deuteronomy 30:19.** I call heaven and earth to witness against you today that I have set before you life and death, blessings and curses. Choose life so that you and your descendants may live.

_____

_____

_____

_____

_____

_____

_____

_____

_____

_____

_____

_____

KEY

# 2

# Admit It! Part 1

Read pages 21–45 in *Think and Eat Yourself Smart* and watch the key 2 video.

1. *Today, the McDonald's logo is more recognizable than the Christian cross.* What are the implications of this? What does this say about our food system? Or our society?

_____

_____

_____

_____

_____

_____

_____

_____

_____

2. *Throughout our history, human beings have survived, and thrived, on a diversity of diets.* What kinds of diets? What does this mean for the way we eat today? Can we adapt to different diets?

_____

_____

_____

_____

3. *Despite the apparent diversity of foodstuffs in our grocery stores, restaurants, and homes, many of the products available for purchase today are industrially manufactured "food-like products," as journalist and activist Michael Pollan calls them.* What are these food-like products? What is the MAD? How is the MAD different from *real* food? What is *real* food?

_____

_____

_____

_____

4. *If there has been one consistent theme across the research I have done for this book, it is that our food systems are wired for love.* What does this statement mean? How are our food systems wired for love?

_____

_____

_____

_____

5. *Many of the best chefs source local, organically grown foods not necessarily for their nutritional benefit but for their wholesome and rich flavor—good nutrition and good flavor are inseparable.* Have you found this in your own life? Why do you think *real* food tastes so good (think of the difference between a store-bought tomato and a homegrown tomato)?

_____

_____

_____

_____

6. *The terms* organic *and* conventional *are controversial and have many interpretations.* What is the difference between organic and conventional agriculture? Are the differences always clear-cut? Is organic agriculture always healthy? Do these stipulations apply to meat production as well?

_____

_____

_____

_____

7. *The word* organic *has taken on an almost religious significance with consumers, yet here is a subtle trap: organic foods can also be refined, preserved, and highly processed.* Have you fallen into this trap? Why is it important to not just trust the label "organic"?

_____

_____

_____

_____

8. *Shipping foods over long distances drains the ability of these foods to truly nourish us.* How so? Why is it important to eat local foods? What does "fresh" food mean? How is this different from preserved or shipped food? How can preservatives be dangerous?

_____

_____

_____

_____

_____

9. *Efficiency and affordability are often traps in themselves, with costs that are not apparent in the purchasing price of many modern foods.* How so? What are these hidden costs?

_____

_____

_____

_____

_____

10. *The architectural layout of the modern supermarket, designed to influence our food choices, poses a threat to our health.* How so? How is the supermarket designed to influence your choices?

_____

_____

_____

_____

_____

11. *We use an "agro-ecological" measuring stick to define* real *food.* What does agro-ecological mean? How is it different from just eating organic? How does this relate to conscious consumerism?

_____

_____

_____

_____

12. *God created a natural world that is characterized by incredible diversity.* Can you think of examples of this diversity? Why is this diversity important?

_____

_____

_____

_____

13. *Food monocultures, such as corn, soy, or wheat, and the factory farming of animals both focus on the mass production of a single species and are removing the delicate ecological balance found in diversity.* What is a monoculture? What are the effects of a monoculture? What are the dominant monocultures in agriculture today?

_____

_____

_____

_____

14. *The modern food industry has taken animals off the farm and placed them in industrial facilities called CAFOs, Concentrated Animal Feeding Operations.* How do CAFOs impact the environment? How do they impact our health, the health of the animals, or the health of the workers?

_____

_____

_____

_____

15. *Human trafficking is a dominant issue in agriculture, both within the United States and globally.* How so? Why is this the case? What is the relationship between trafficking and cheap food?

_____

_____

_____

_____

16. *The monetary cost of cheap meat, like that of mass-produced bread and other foodstuffs, does not reflect the true price paid to bring it to our plates.* What are the hidden costs of cheap meat?

_____

_____

_____

_____

17. *The MAD is aptly named, since it is high in refined sugar, salt, and saturated fat, which are added to make the processed food-stuffs edible and attractive.* Why is the MAD mad? What are the effects of processed sugar, salt, and fat?

_____

_____

_____

_____

18. *The MAD is not just an American problem. It is one of the United States' most successful, and ubiquitous, exports.* How has America exported the MAD? What are the effects of this export? What is the obesity epidemic?

_____

_____

_____

_____

19. *In the globalized world we live in today, what we buy for dinner has international repercussions—there is a definite "butterfly effect" associated with our food choices.* What is this butterfly effect? Why is what we choose to eat important? How does this relate to loving our neighbor?

_____

_____

_____

_____

*Think and Eat Yourself Smart* focuses on the state of our current food system. Discuss the following verses in light of this theme.

1. **Matthew 5:48.** Be perfect, therefore, as your heavenly Father is perfect.
2. **Matthew 25:23.** You have been trustworthy in a few things, I will put you in charge of many things; enter into the joy of your master.
3. **Psalm 139:14.** I praise you, for I am fearfully and wonderfully made.

_____

_____

_____

_____

_____

_____

_____

_____

_____

_____

_____

_____

_____

_____

# KEY
# 3

## Admit It! Part 2

Read pages 46–59 in *Think and Eat Yourself Smart* and watch the key 3 video.

1. *Part of the strong allure of our industrial food system is its convenience, a factor that has greatly contributed to its global success.* Why do you think that convenience is so alluring? Does convenience determine what you eat on a daily basis? Why? Do you think this is a healthy way to eat?

   _____

   _____

   _____

   _____

2. *In 1937, George Orwell said, "We may find in the long run that tinned food is a deadlier weapon than the machine-gun."* Do you think this statement is true? If yes, how so? If no, why?

_____

_____

_____

_____

_____

_____

3. *The truth is that none of us can afford the true price of fol-lowing the MAD: its low cost is a dangerous illusion.* Why is cheap food a dangerous illusion? Are the true costs of the food reflected in its price tag?

_____

_____

_____

_____

_____

4. *Millions of people cannot afford real, whole foods, which is one of the principal tragedies of our dysfunctional food system—a system that has "forgotten to feed people well."* Is there a way to help people who cannot afford to buy *real* food? How can you help people who cannot afford to purchase *real* food? Does buying *real* food help people who cannot afford it? How so?

_____

_____

_____

_____

_____

5. *It is essential that we not only "vote with our votes" to demand official changes in food policy and support government officials who are trying to change our current food system but also "vote with our forks."* How can we "vote with our votes" for a better food system? How can we "vote with our forks" for a fairer system of food production?

_____

_____

_____

_____

_____

_____

6. *Large corporations spend millions of dollars on research annually, calculating the precise amount of fat, sugar, and salt that will satisfy our taste buds and keep us coming back for more, regardless of the health consequences.* How do large corporations do this? Is this true in your own life or the life of someone you know? How addictive are processed foods?

_____

_____

_____

_____

7. *One of the leading centers of food research in the United States, Monell Chemical Senses Center, has performed experiments on young children, feeding them various sugary foods to calculate their "bliss point," the level at which their desire for sugar is at*

*its climax*. What is the purpose of this experiment? What are other ways large corporations market junk food to children? Is this ethical? Would you allow your own child or another child you know to participate in this experiment? How does junk food affect children?

_____

_____

_____

_____

_____

8. *Our current industrial food system has created an environment that essentially floods our senses, adults and children alike, with the message of "eat more" unhealthy, processed foods.* Can you think of examples of this? Is this true in your own life or the life of someone you know? How is this message of eating more affecting our health and the health of our environment?

_____

_____

_____

_____

_____

_____

9. *We are bombarded with phrases like "high in Vitamin C," "full of great antioxidants," "low fat," and a "great source of omega fatty acids," but these are largely marketing devices supported by unhealthy scientific reductionism.* Why should we be wary when we see statements like these? Why is this a

form of reductionism? How does the modern food industry divorce foods from the context of real life?

_____

_____

_____

_____

_____

10. *Medicine is ultimately medicine, whether it is man-made or found in nature, and there are many things in nature that can harm us, such as poisonous plants and fungi.* Are supplements medicine? Why should we be careful of taking too many supplements?

_____

_____

_____

_____

11. *Exercise, however, can never replace an unhealthy diet; it is not a magic bullet that will allow you to eat whatever you feel like without any consequences.* Do you think this statement is true? If yes, how so? If no, why? Is this true in your own life? What do you think is a healthy exercise-diet balance?

_____

_____

_____

_____

## DISCUSSION

*Think and Eat Yourself Smart* focuses on the state of our current food system. Discuss the following verses in light of this theme.

1. **Matthew 5:16.** In the same way, let your light shine before others, so that they may see your good works and give glory to your Father in heaven.

2. **1 Corinthians 10:31.** So, whether you eat or drink, or whatever you do, do everything for the glory of God.

3. **Mark 12:31.** You shall love your neighbor as yourself.

_____

_____

_____

_____

_____

_____

_____

_____

_____

_____

_____

_____

_____

_____

_____

_____

# 4

## Admit It! Part 3

Read pages 60–80 in *Think and Eat Yourself Smart* and watch the key 4 video.

1. *By controlling the supply chains, large food corporations rule the economic roost.* What is the nature of this control? How does it affect us? Are the effects worldwide?

_____

_____

_____

_____

2. *Access to healthier foods such as fresh fruit and vegetables is limited by price manipulations generated by government subsidization of foods like corn, soy, and wheat.* Is the cheap food in our stores and restaurants naturally cheap? How is the food system manipulated by subsidies? How does this prevent people

from being able to afford *real* food? How does this affect our health?

_____

_____

_____

_____

_____

3. *Millions of Americans, and particularly people in inner-city neighborhoods, live in "food deserts."* What are food deserts? Do you have any food deserts near you? Do you live in a food desert?

_____

_____

_____

_____

_____

4. *Unfortunately, government officials are as likely to have a relationship with the food industry as they are to police it.* What is the relationship like between the government and food corporations? What is a revolving door? How do you think this impacts laws on food production? Is this something that should concern us?

_____

_____

_____

_____

5. *Smaller, more biologically diverse family farms cannot compete with the power of these large food corporations.* Why? Has this happened where you live? What are the implications of large-scale factory farming?

_____

_____

_____

_____

_____

6. *Today, we could feed the world's starving with a percentage of the food that is thrown away throughout the world.* What is the global waste scandal? Are you guilty of wasting food?

_____

_____

_____

_____

_____

7. *Genetically engineered food production [is] otherwise known as recombinant DNA technology.* What is recombinant DNA technology? How are GM (genetically modified) foods used today?

_____

_____

_____

_____

_____

8. *To argue that GM foods are completely safe is to deny that there are many things we have yet to learn about genes, let alone the way genes react in an organism within our multifaceted ecosystems.* Should we blindly trust the science behind GM foods? How can GM foods potentially harm us?

_____

_____

_____

_____

_____

9. *The potential risks of GM food production are not limited to human health.* What are these other risks? How can GM foods affect the environment?

_____

_____

_____

_____

_____

10. *Today, we have enough food to feed the world.* How so? Why do people still starve and suffer from malnutrition?

_____

_____

_____

_____

_____

11. *The growing body of research on agro-ecological farming methods offers some exciting possibilities.* What are these exciting possibilities? How can this type of farming potentially feed the world?

_____

_____

_____

_____

_____

_____

12. *Rather than trying to change what God has given us in nature, a far better use of science in our food system is science that devises ingenious solutions that imitate God's creation.* How can we do this? What is biomimicry?

_____

_____

_____

_____

_____

_____

## DISCUSSION

*Think and Eat Yourself Smart* focuses on the state of our current food system. Discuss the following verses in light of this theme.

1. **Genesis 2:15**. The LORD God took the man and put him in the garden of Eden to till it and keep it.
2. **Psalm 24:1–2**. The earth is the LORD's and all that is in it, the world, and those who live in it; for he has founded it on the seas, and established it on the rivers.
3. **John 1:3**. All things came into being through him, and without him not one thing came into being.

_____

_____

_____

_____

_____

_____

_____

_____

_____

_____

_____

_____

_____

_____

# KEY

# 5

## Quit It! Part 1

Read pages 83–115 in *Think and Eat Yourself Smart* and watch the key 5 video.

1. *The mindset behind the meal—the thinking behind the meal— plays a dominant role in the process of human food-related health issues.* How so? Why is thinking so important when it comes to eating? Is this true in your own life? How do you believe thinking differently can improve the way you eat?

   _____

   _____

   _____

   _____

2. *If we do not have a healthy mind, then nothing else in our life will be healthy, including our eating habits.* Why? Can you think of examples in your own life? Do you think a *real*-food

lifestyle is possible without changing the way we think about food?

_____

_____

_____

_____

_____

3. *Although your brain is only 2 percent of the weight of your body, it consumes 20 percent of the total energy (oxygen) and 65 percent of the glucose.* How important is eating healthy for proper brain function? How well can you think and learn when you eat the Modern American Diet? Can you think of examples in your own life?

_____

_____

_____

_____

_____

4. *Those of us who can afford to purchase better quality food, once we understand how dysfunctional our current food system is, have a responsibility to change the way we eat.* Do you think so? If yes, why? If no, why not?

_____

_____

_____

_____

5. *As a culture, we have become so accustomed to our current, global MAD food system that it has become a part of our nonconscious minds.* Do you think about where the food you eat came from? If yes, how often? Why? And, if no, can you think of a reason why you don't think about how your food came to be on your plate? Do you think it is important to be aware of where your food came from?

_____

_____

_____

_____

_____

_____

6. *Many individuals do not know, or do not want to acknowledge, how dysfunctional our food system actually is.* Do you think this statement is true? If yes, why? If no, why not? Is this true in your own life?

_____

_____

_____

_____

_____

_____

7. *Our ultimate goals should therefore be a healthy diet and a lifestyle that nourishes and sustains us, not a supermodel body that is defined by superficial cultural standards.* Do you think that many people only think about food when it comes to losing

weight? Is this true in your own life? How does this type of thinking limit us when it comes to food and healthy living?

_____

_____

_____

_____

8. *When you are thinking, choosing, and forming thoughts or memories, your mind is "in action."* What does this statement mean? How does it relate to the Geodesic Information Processing Theory? How does a mind "in action" relate to neuroplasticity, the ability of the brain to change?

_____

_____

_____

_____

9. *You literally wire thoughts into your brain, thereby transforming the biological landscape of your brain.* How so? Why is this important?

_____

_____

_____

_____

10. *The nonconscious metacognitive level of the mind is incredibly extensive.* What is this level of the mind? Why is it important? How does it relate to the "I-factor"?

_____

_____

_____

_____

_____

11. *The conscious level of the mind is responsible for roughly 1–10 percent of our mind's activity.* What is this level of the mind? Why is it important?

_____

_____

_____

_____

_____

12. *We have the ability, with our conscious mind, to change and reconceptualize embedded memories.* Why is this important when it comes to eating? How does this relate to the Quantum Zeno Effect (QZE)? How does this relate to learning?

_____

_____

_____

_____

_____

13. *[The] senses are the bridge between the external world that we inhabit and the internal world of our mind.* Why are the

senses important? Why is it important to watch what we allow in (and out) through our senses?

_____

_____

_____

_____

14. *Marketing campaigns firehose information into your conscious mind through your five senses.* How can these campaigns influence our food decisions? Can you think of an example in your own life? How can we control the impact of food marketing campaigns?

_____

_____

_____

_____

15. *When it comes to food, our fast-paced modern lifestyles have produced the mindset of "I am too busy to cook, and convenient foods at least give me a little bit of time to do what I want. I just need a break."* Do you find that this is true in your own life? How can our busy schedules affect our thinking and eating patterns? How have we become a "fast-food nation"? Is it important to take time off to eat well? How do social media and TV play into our "hurry sickness"?

_____

_____

_____

_____

16. *As a society, we should be especially concerned about the impact of food marketing on our children.* Why? How does food marketing to children impact their mental and physical health and their future?

_____

_____

_____

_____

17. *Although policies and regulations have been introduced to control food marketing, they are often flawed.* How so? How can we control food marketing?

_____

_____

_____

_____

_____

18. *We have to choose to process this information, or create a mindset/habit in our nonconscious minds based on the information we receive on a daily basis through our five senses.* What does this statement mean? How does it relate to the power of choice and the ability to choose a healthy, *real*-food lifestyle?

_____

_____

_____

_____

_____

## DISCUSSION

*Think and Eat Yourself Smart* focuses on the state of our current food system. Discuss the following verses in light of this theme.

1. **2 Corinthians 10:5.** We take every thought captive to obey Christ.
2. **1 Corinthians 16:13.** Keep alert, stand firm in your faith, be courageous, be strong.
3. **Romans 8:37.** In all these things we are more than conquerors through him who loved us.

_____

_____

_____

_____

_____

_____

_____

_____

_____

_____

_____

_____

_____

_____

_____

_____

KEY

# 6

# Quit It! Part 2

Read pages 116–53 in *Think and Eat Yourself Smart* and watch the key 6 video.

1. *The act of eating is not just a biological function for survival.* How so? Why is eating about more than just survival? Is this true in your own life?

_____

_____

_____

_____

_____

_____

2. *Our gastrointestinal (GI) tract is very sensitive to our emotions.* How so? What is the gut-brain connection? How does eating

affect this connection? Can you think of examples in your own life? How does emotional eating affect this connection?

_____

_____

_____

_____

_____

3. *Digestive functioning even affects our sleeping patterns.* How so? Is this true in your own life?

_____

_____

_____

_____

_____

4. *The gastrointestinal (GI) system is controlled by the enteric nervous system (ENS), often called the "second brain."* What is the ENS? Why is it important?

_____

_____

_____

_____

5. *Our emotions impact not only the way our body digests food but also our choices—before our meal even enters our mouths!*

How so? Why is it so important to have a good attitude when it comes to all aspects of eating?

_____

_____

_____

_____

_____

6. *When we eat reactively, that is, without deliberately examining the mindsets embedded in our nonconscious minds, we increase our risk for making unhealthy food choices.* How so? Is this true in your own life?

_____

_____

_____

_____

_____

7. *All the structures of our brains and bodies are wired for love.* What does this statement mean? Why is this important when it comes to our eating habits?

_____

_____

_____

_____

_____

8. *We live in a world that tends toward intellectual reductionism.* How has this affected the way we eat food? Or the way we view our relationship with food and health?

_____

_____

_____

_____

9. *One aid to disciplining the mind is fasting.* How can fasting help with our mental and physical health? What are some of the benefits of fasting?

_____

_____

_____

_____

10. *The unscrupulous use of brain imaging by media outlets, companies, university press offices, and many researchers seems to offer us physical proof that everything from obesity to murder originates from a brain that is imbalanced or diseased. These visual pictures are misleading when it comes to where the responsibility lies for our health.* How so? Can you think of examples of the use of brain imaging? Why can this be misleading?

_____

_____

_____

_____

11. *Today, there is a massive split in the world of neuroscience.* What is this split? How do different views of the mind affect our perception of the mind, brain, and body? What is a neuro-centric worldview? How can it have a negative effect when it comes to our health?

_____

_____

_____

_____

_____

12. *Where the mind goes, the brain and body follow.* How so? Is the mind powerful?

_____

_____

_____

_____

_____

13. *Many diet plans today are principally based on behavioral changes.* Why does this approach fall short of creating real, lasting change when it comes to what we eat? What is a better way of approaching the issue of diet and food choices?

_____

_____

_____

_____

_____

14. *When we discipline, or renew, our minds, we change how we think about eating, thereby changing the framework of our food choices.* Why is this a better way to change the way we think about and eat food?

_____

_____

_____

_____

15. *Change is not instant.* Why does it take time to change the way we eat? How much time? Why is healthy eating and thinking a *lifestyle*?

_____

_____

_____

_____

16. *What we choose to eat affects not only our health but our children's health as well.* How so? Is this true in your own life?

_____

_____

_____

_____

17. *One category of self-destructive food behavior is eating disorders.* How do eating disorders start in the mind? Are they thought disorders or diseases? Why? Can people quit food addictions like eating disorders by changing the way they think?

_____

_____

_____

_____

18. *Walter Willet, chair of Harvard's department of nutrition and also one of the single most cited nutritionists today, points his finger directly at the food companies when it comes to today's food system.* How do these food companies manipulate what we eat and create food addictions? Can we overcome these food addictions? Is food addiction a disease?

_____

_____

_____

_____

19. *Our brain's reward circuits fire up a neurophysiological response par excellence when we think and eat in a healthy way.* How are we designed to be addicted to love? How does this relate to how we think about and eat food? How can we use our thinking to fight the machinations of large food corporations?

_____

_____

_____

_____

20. *Epigenetics examines how environments regulate gene activity and expression as a response to both internal and external signals.* What does this statement mean? Why is this so important

when it comes to what we choose to eat and how we choose to think about food? How does our environment affect our biology? What is the relationship between our choices, our thoughts, and our genetics?

_____

_____

_____

_____

_____

21. *God has set up a complex and beautiful interplay between us, our biology, and our environments.* How so? Why is it important to look at food holistically? How does food affect the environment around our cells?

_____

_____

_____

_____

_____

22. *As Michael Pollan says, "You are what you eat eats."* Why are we "what we eat eats"? What does this quote mean?

_____

_____

_____

_____

_____

23. *Our food choices are not the only epigenetic legacies we leave to our children.* How so? What kind of legacy are you leaving, or will you be leaving, for your children?

_____

_____

_____

_____

_____

## DISCUSSION

*Think and Eat Yourself Smart* focuses on the state of our current food system. Discuss the following verses in light of this theme.

1. **1 Corinthians 10:31.** So, whether you eat or drink, or whatever you do, do everything for the glory of God.
2. **Matthew 6:33.** But strive first for the kingdom of God and his righteousness, and all these things will be given to you as well.
3. **2 Timothy 1:7.** For God did not give us a spirit of cowardice, but rather a spirit of power and of love and of self-discipline.

_____

_____

_____

_____

_____

_____

_____

_____

_____

_____

_____

_____

_____

_____

_____

KEY

# 7

## Quit It! Part 3

Read pages 154–210 in *Think and Eat Yourself Smart* and watch the key 7 video.

1. *The right protein choices positively affect the environment around our cells, and thus our health.* How so? What are healthy protein choices?

_____

_____

_____

_____

_____

_____

_____

_____

_____

_____

2. *Your brain thrives on good-quality protein sources.* How so? Have you found that this is true in your own life? What happens when you don't eat good-quality proteins?

_____

_____

_____

_____

_____

3. *Of the twenty amino acids needed for proper construction of proteins, eight (or nine, for children) are called essential amino acids, since the body cannot synthesize or make these for itself.* What are these amino acids used for? How do we get these amino acids?

_____

_____

_____

_____

4. *Another important point to note about meat is how much muscle meat we consume, and the impact this has on our bodies.* What are muscle meats? Why is it important not to eat too much muscle meat? What are alternatives to muscle meat? Why should we have a nose-to-tail approach if we eat meat?

_____

_____

_____

_____

5. *Many individuals today equate the consumption of animal protein sources with cholesterol levels and a higher risk of mortality.* Why do people think this? What is wrong with the science behind this statement? Do we need cholesterol?

_____

_____

_____

_____

6. *One of the key figures behind the diet-heart hypothesis that dietary cholesterol can lead to cardiovascular disease was Ancel Keys.* Who was Ancel Keys? What was his hypothesis? How has his hypothesis affected us today? Where did his hypothesis go wrong?

_____

_____

_____

_____

_____

7. *Your body needs fat for all its processes, as does your brain.* Why do we need fat? What are good sources of fat? What fats should we avoid?

_____

_____

_____

_____

_____

8. *The key is not to focus solely on individual pieces of the puzzle like saturated fat or cholesterol.* Why? What should we focus on?

_____

_____

_____

_____

9. *MAD sugar, the refined and processed sugar so many of us consume today, disrupts the intricately balanced environments in our brain and body.* How so? What is MAD sugar? What contains MAD sugar? Why are these types of processed sugars "empty calories"? How are they different from the natural sugars found in whole foods like fruit and honey?

_____

_____

_____

_____

10. *Sugar eventually ends up in the pleasure centers in our brains, such as the orbital frontal cortex, where we consciously experience the pull of the "sugar rush."* How does this relate to sugar addiction? How is MAD sugar addictive? Can we overcome sugar addiction?

_____

_____

_____

_____

11. *Glucose and fructose are metabolized differently in the body.* How so? Why is this important when it comes to the food we eat? What is the balance between glucose and fructose in processed, MAD sugars? What is this balance in natural sugars?

_____

_____

_____

_____

_____

12. *The brain's many structures and circuits work on the principle of connectivity.* How so? Why is this important when it comes to the food we eat?

_____

_____

_____

_____

_____

13. *The manufacturing process for HFCS is different than that of table sugar.* What is HFCS? Why is it so unhealthy? How is it produced?

_____

_____

_____

_____

_____

14. *Eating a diet high in processed and refined foods can also cause resistance to the anabolic hormone insulin, which in turn can contribute to the onset of chronic diseases and even early death.* How so? Why is this so dangerous?

_____

_____

_____

_____

_____

15. *The number of people with Alzheimer's disease is projected to increase fourfold over the next forty years, reaching approximately fourteen million by 2050.* Why is this so alarming? What is the relationship between our mental health, our memory, and the food we eat?

_____

_____

_____

_____

_____

16. *By making gluten the root of all dietary evils, we once again step into reductionist thinking, where one ingredient or chemical is blamed for most of the woes of mankind, and where the small subset of those genuinely afflicted is made to represent the larger population.* How so? Why is "gluten free" turning into a diet fad? Are most people allergic to gluten? How is gluten intolerance different from celiac disease?

_____

_____

_____

_____

_____

_____

17. *Our MAD food system has dramatically changed the grains we eat and the way we eat grains.* How so? How has this contributed to the rising number of people who are intolerant to gluten?

_____

_____

_____

_____

_____

18. *We cannot think good food thoughts without sleep, and we can't digest the food we eat well without sleep.* Why? Have you found that this is true in your own life? How can a lack of sleep cause us to eat more processed foods or overeat?

_____

_____

_____

_____

19. *We are designed to move, for the sake of both the brain and body.* Why is exercise so important? How can exercise complement a *real*-food lifestyle?

_____

_____

_____

_____

_____

_____

20. *Our overall ability to think and understand through intellectualizing and shifting through our thoughts is improved with exercise, regardless of our age.* How so? Have you found that this is true in your own life? What is BDNF, and why is it important? How does it relate to exercise?

_____

_____

_____

_____

_____

_____

## DISCUSSION

*Think and Eat Yourself Smart* focuses on the state of our current food system. Discuss the following verses in light of this theme.

1. **1 Corinthians 6:19–20.** Or do you not know that your body is a temple of the Holy Spirit within you, which you have from God, and that you are not your own? For you were bought with a price; therefore glorify God in your body.

2. **Philippians 4:19.** And my God will fully satisfy every need of yours according to his riches in glory in Christ Jesus.

3. **Colossians 3:17.** And whatever you do, in word or deed, do everything in the name of the Lord Jesus, giving thanks to God the Father through him.

_____

_____

_____

_____

_____

_____

_____

_____

_____

_____

_____

_____

_____

KEY

# 8

# **Beat It! Part 1**

Read pages 213–23 (through Tip 5) in *Think and Eat Yourself Smart* and watch the key 8 video.

1. *It is not so much about eating or avoiding specific foods for your mental and physical health; it is all about thinking right and eating real food.* Why? What is the best way to eat food?

_____

_____

_____

_____

_____

_____

_____

_____

_____

2. *The key is to renew the way you think about food and thereby renew your food choices.* How does changing the way we think about food help us change the way we eat food?

_____

_____

_____

_____

_____

3. *I am not offering an overnight, quick-fix, magic-bullet, or reductionist solution.* Why do these quick solutions so often fail when it comes to developing and maintaining a healthy lifestyle?

_____

_____

_____

_____

_____

4. *Our brains and bodies function well when we eat* real *food.* How so? What is *real* food? Can you think of some real-life examples? How does eating bad food affect the way you think?

_____

_____

_____

_____

_____

5. *You are, and you become, what you think.* What does this statement mean? What are some ways you can control your thinking when it comes to food?

_____

_____

_____

_____

_____

6. *We have to understand that choice is real and will have real consequences.* How are choices real? Why are they so powerful? How can you control your choices?

_____

_____

_____

_____

_____

7. *The brain and mind are separate, and the mind controls the brain.* What does this statement mean? Why is this so important? How can you use the power of your mind to change your eating patterns?

_____

_____

_____

_____

_____

8. *It takes around twenty-one days to rewire neural pathways and begin building a new way of thinking about food and forty-two days (another two sets of twenty-one days, for a total of sixty-three days) to establish a new habit.* How can we develop new eating habits? Why is it so important to give ourselves time when developing new eating habits? How are you going to start developing better thinking and eating patterns?

_____

_____

_____

_____

_____

9. *The GI tract is very sensitive to our emotions and works closely with the hypothalamus in the brain, which responds to our emotions and the feeling of satiety.* Why is it important to be aware of our emotions before eating? How can emotional eating impact our health? What is deliberative eating? How can you start eating more deliberatively?

_____

_____

_____

_____

_____

## DISCUSSION

*Think and Eat Yourself Smart* focuses on the state of our current food system. Discuss the following verses in light of this theme.

1. **1 Corinthians 9:25.** Athletes exercise self-control in all things; they do it to receive a perishable wreath, but we an imperishable one.

2. **Galatians 5:16.** Live by the Spirit, I say, and do not gratify the desires of the flesh.

3. **Proverbs 25:28.** Like a city breached, without walls, is one who lacks self-control.

_____

_____

_____

_____

_____

_____

_____

_____

_____

_____

_____

_____

_____

_____

_____

_____

# KEY
# 9

## Beat It! Part 2

Read pages 223–34 (starting at Tip 6) in *Think and Eat Yourself Smart* and watch the key 9 video.

1. *There is no one particular way of eating that works for everyone.* Must all people eat the same foods? Why is it important to listen to our bodies when eating food and to be careful of diet fads?

   _____

   _____

   _____

   _____

2. *When purchasing any food item, make sure it is* real *food insofar as possible, not a food-like product.* What are good places to buy *real* food? Have you found places that sell *real* food near you, or good farm-to-table restaurants? Why is it important

to have a diverse diet? Can you start growing or raising some of your own foods?

_____

_____

_____

_____

3. *As stewards of God's creation, we glorify him when we steward the earth's resources well and we eat food that nourishes us and glorifies the creation of our own bodies.* How does the principle of stewardship apply to eating? How can you become a better steward of creation?

_____

_____

_____

_____

4. *Often, diet books are so concerned about what you eat that they do not explain how you should prepare these meals to preserve the most nutrients possible.* What are some healthy cooking methods? How can you cook healthier in your own life?

_____

_____

_____

_____

5. *Our fast-paced modern lifestyles have produced the mindset of "I am too busy to sit down to a home-cooked meal."* What

are some healthy ways of eating food? What is *hara hachi bu*? How can you eat food better?

_____

_____

_____

_____

_____

6. *The brain and the gut are connected in many things, including sleep and schedules.* Why is sleep so important when it comes to what we eat? How can you improve your sleeping schedule?

_____

_____

_____

_____

7. *Eat less, move more: we have all heard this saying at some point in our lives.* Why is exercise so important? How do you like to work out? Can you improve your exercise regimen?

_____

_____

_____

_____

8. *Your mind makes exercise much more effective.* How so? How can you use your mind when you exercise?

_____

_____

_____

_____

*Think and Eat Yourself Smart* focuses on the state of our current food system. Discuss the following verses in light of this theme.

1. **Genesis 2:15.** The LORD God took the man and put him in the garden of Eden to till it and keep it.
2. **1 Corinthians 4:2.** It is required of stewards that they be found trustworthy.
3. **Matthew 6:13.** And do not bring us to the time of trial, but rescue us from the evil one.

_____

_____

_____

_____

_____

_____

_____

_____

_____

_____

_____

_____

# Conclusion

Congratulations! You are well on your way to thinking *and* eating yourself smart!

When it comes to eating, do not fall for quick tricks, fancy programs, or weight-loss gimmicks. There is no simple or quick program that will give you purpose and help you succeed in life. It takes good, old-fashioned hard work and a habit of deep, intentional thinking to change the way you think about and eat food—but the effort is well worth it!

Now that you have opened your mind to a new, healthy way of approaching food and have started removing unhealthy foods and habits from your everyday life, you have entered a culinary world bursting with magnificent smells, tastes, sights, sounds, and feelings that will bring joy to both your mind and your stomach!

As you carry on in your journey, never forget how important the mind is when it comes to eating! There will always be a plethora of complicated messages and marketing advertisements telling you what to eat, but if your mind is healthy, you can stand strong in your decision to live a healthy, happy life. If your mind is strong, nourished by good thoughts and *real* food, you can admit, quit, and beat the MAD food system for good.

The choice is yours!

# Recommended Reading List

Robinson, Jo. *Eating on the Wild Side: The Missing Link to Optimum Health*. New York: Little, Brown and Company, 2014.

Pollan, Michael. *The Omnivore's Dilemma: A Natural History of Four Meals*. New York: Penguin Press, 2006.

———. *Food Rules: An Eater's Manual*. New York: Penguin Books, 2014.

———. *In Defense of Food: An Eater's Manifesto*. London: Penguin Books, 2009.

Salatin, Joel. *Folks, This Ain't Normal: A Farmer's Advice for Happier Hens, Healthier People, and a Better World*. New York: Center Street, 2012.

Schlosser, Eric. *Fast Food Nation: The Dark Side of the All-American Meal*. Boston: Mariner Books/Houghton Mifflin Harcourt, 2012.

Moss, Michael. *Salt Sugar Fat: How the Food Giants Hooked Us*. New York: Random House, 2014.

Nestle, Marion. *Food Politics: How the Food Industry Influences Nutrition and Health*. Berkeley: University of California Press, 2013.

Gustafson, Ellen. *We the Eaters: If We Change Dinner, We Can Change the World*. Emmaus: Rodale, 2014.

Allen, Will, and Charles Wilson. *The Good Food Revolution: Growing Healthy Food, People, and Communities.* New York: Gotham Books, 2013.

Stuart, Tristram. *Waste: Uncovering the Global Food Scandal.* London: W.W. Norton, 2009.

Patel, Raj. *Stuffed and Starved: The Hidden Battle for the World Food System.* Brooklyn: Melville House, 2014.

Barber, Dan. *The Third Plate: Field Notes on the Future of Food.* New York: Penguin Books, 2014.

Berry, Wendell. *The Unsettling of America: Culture & Agriculture.* San Francisco: Sierra Club Books, 1997.

Bittman, Mark. *A Bone to Pick: The Good and Bad News about Food, with Wisdom, Insights, and Advice on Diets, Food Safety, GMOs, Farming, and More.* New York: Clarkson Potter, 2015.

Shiva, Vandana. *Earth Democracy: Justice, Sustainability, and Peace.* London: Zed Books Ltd., 2006.

Hesterman, Oran B. *Fair Food: Growing a Healthy, Sustainable Food System for All.* New York: PublicAffairs, 2012.

Buettner, Dan. *The Blue Zone: Lessons for Living Longer from the People Who've Lived the Longest.* Washington, DC: National Geographic, 2012.

Benyus, Janine M. *Biomimicry: Innovation Inspired by Nature.* New York: HarperCollins, 2009.

White, Courtney. *Grass, Soil, Hope: A Journey through Carbon Country.* White River Junction, VT: Chelsea Green, 2014.

**Dr. Caroline Leaf** is a communication pathologist and cognitive neuroscientist. Since the early 1980s, she has researched the mind-brain connection, the nature of mental health, and the formation of memory. She was one of the first in her field to study how the brain can change (neuroplasticity). Her passion is to help people see how the power of the mind can change the brain and how the link between science and spirituality can help them control their thoughts and emotions, learn how to think and learn, and find their sense of purpose in life. She is the author of *Switch On Your Brain*, *Think and Eat Yourself Smart*, *The Perfect You*, and *Think, Learn, Succeed*, among many other books and journal articles, and her videos, podcasts, and TV episodes have reached millions globally. She currently teaches at academic, medical, and neuroscience conferences; churches; and to various audiences around the world. Dr. Leaf and her husband, Mac, live with their four children in Dallas and Los Angeles.

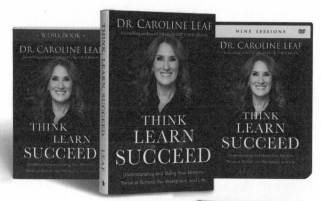
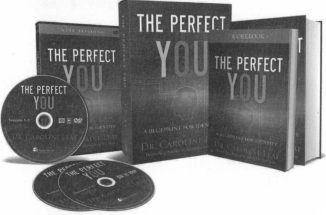
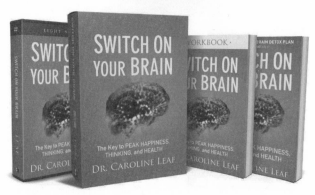
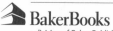